# ALL YOU WANTED TO KNOW ABOUT
# *Headache*

*Edited by*
**Dr Savitri Ramaiah**

New Dawn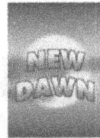

NEW DAWN
a division of Sterling Publishers (P) Ltd.
L-10, Green Park Extension, New Delhi-110016
Ph.: 6191784, 6191785, 6191023  Fax: 91-11-6190028
E-mail: ghai@nde.vsnl.net.in
Internet: http://www.sterlingpublishers.com

*Headache*
©1999, Sterling Publishers Private Limited
ISBN  978 81 207 9467 2
Reprint 2000

*Published by* Sterling Publishers Pvt. Ltd., New Delhi-110016.
*Lasertypeset by* Vikas Compographics, New Delhi-110029.
*Printed at* Shagun Composer, New Delhi-110029

Information for this series, has been provided by *Health Update*, a monthly bulletin of the Society for Health Education and Learning Packages. The Update is intended to provide you with knowledge to adopt preventive measures and cooperate with the doctor during illness for better outcome of treatment.

Contributors

**ALLOPATHY**
Dr. L. Krishnamurthy
*(Profassor and Head, Department of Neurology, J.J.M. Medical College)*

**AYURVEDA**
Dr. V.N. Pandey
*(Director, Central Council for Research in Ayurveda and Siddha, New Delhi)*

**HOMOEOPATHY**
Dr. V. K. Khanna
*(Principal, Nehru Homoeopathic College, Delhi)*

Dr. Poonam Jain
*(Consultant Homoeopathy, Delhi)*

**NATURE CURE**
Dr. Sambhashiva Rao
*(Former Chief Medical Officer, Institute of Naturopathy, Bangalore)*

# Preface

*All You Wanted to Know About* is an easy-to-read reference series put together by *Health Update* and assisted by a team of medical experts who offer the latest perspectives on body health.

Each book in the series enhances your knowledge on a particular health issue. It makes you an active participant by giving multiple perspectives to choose from — allopathy, acupuncture, ayurveda, homoeopathy, nature cure and unani.

This book is intended as a home adviser but does not substitute a doctor.

The opinions are those of the contributors, and the publisher holds no responsibility.

# Contents

# Introduction

Headache, can be defined as discomfort or pain in the head. Tension, migraine, cluster, cervicogenic, after injury, vascular and effort-induced are some of the different types of headaches. In rare cases the headache may be due to a serious diseases such as bleeding in the space around the brain, fever, increased pressure on the brain, severe hypertension and inflammation of some arteries.

Ayurveda lists diet, life-style, environment, psychological, season and injury as common causes of headache. It is to be noted that only 1% of headaches are serious.

# ALLOPATHY

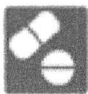

Headache is the term used for discomfort or pain in the head. It could be located anywhere in the area between the forehead in front and the region just above the neck at the back. It is one of the most painful conditions that adversely affects the quality of your life. Headache is not a disease but a symptom. Majority of the headaches are not due to any serious disease.

# How common is headache?

About seventy percent of patients visiting a doctor complain of headache as one of their major problems. Nearly ninety percent of the people have headache at least once in a year. Of these, almost fifty percent are unable to do their normal work during headache. Women are more likely to suffer from the headache as compared to males. This is especially true for migraine headache.

Up to eighty-three percent people take medicines for the headache. However, only about fifty-five percent people with migraine and sixteen percent people with tension headache take treatment from a doctor. Taking medicines without doctor's advice may lead to wrong medication. This in turn can lead to dependence on medicines and more frequent headache. Also, there are many simple non-medicinal measures to control your headache. It is therefore important for you to understand the type of headache you have and then plan effective control measures in consultation with your doctor.

# What are the common types of headache?

In 1988, the International Headache Society defined guidelines for classification of headaches. However, it is not always possible to classify the type of headache. This is because the headache may fulfill more than one criteria for the diagnosis. It is likely that the symptoms may change after some time of your getting recurrent headache. Occasionally the headache changes its characteristics even during one episode.

The common types of headache include tension, migraine, cluster,

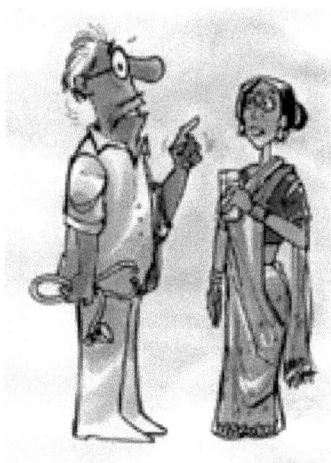

Only one regular patient of headache today. All the others have changed their life-style!

cervicogenic, after injury, vascular and effort-induced. In rare cases the headache may be due to serious diseases such as bleeding in the space around the brain, fever, increased pressure on the brain, severe hypertension and inflammation of some arteries of the brain. Signs, symptoms, causes and treatment for these types of headache are discussed in further chapters.

# Migraine

## What is migraine?

Migraine is a complete disease process and headache is a part of this process. It is important to remember that migraine is **not** just a very severe headache but a *different type of headache*. According to the World Federation of Neurology, migraine is a disorder with recurrent attacks of headache. These headaches differ in intensity, frequency and duration. Most migraine attacks result in pain on one side of the head. These attacks are associated with loss of appetite, nausea, & vomiting. Some neurological symptoms or mood disturbances may be observed before the beginning of a migraine. Women suffer two to three times more often from migraine than men. Most migraines start before the age of forty years.

# What are the causes of migraine?

The exact cause of migraine is not known. Some people have frequent migraine attacks due to *"hereditary factors"*. Adverse environmental conditions precipitate migraine in these people.

*"Serotonin or 5-HT"*, a chemical substance of the brain plays a very important role in migraine. Serotonin is used by nerves for communication. Whenever the nerve endings are stimulated, they

secrete Serotonin. The serotonin links with a special area called a *"receptor"*. Receptors are present all over the body. This link between the serotonin and its receptors results in a specific reaction. Depending on the type of receptor activated by serotonin, there are reactions in the alimentary canal, some blood cells and nerve tissues. In addition to its role in headache, serotonin also affects sleep, blood vessel activity and sexual behaviour. Headache results whenever there is distension of the blood vessels of the brain.

## Fig 1. Mechanism of development of migraine

**Migraine Triggers** ——————→

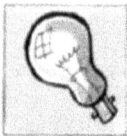
Glare/lights

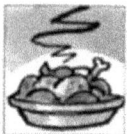
Pungent smell

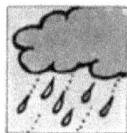
Some foods

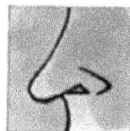
Emotions

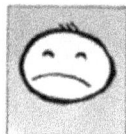
Weather

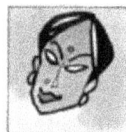
Female hormones

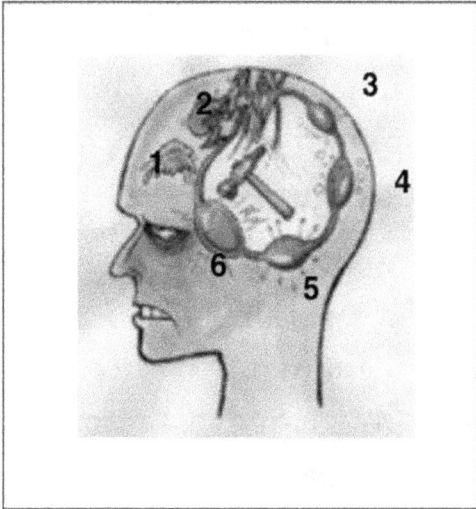

1. Serotonin levels decrease.
2. No regulation of arteries.
3. Blood vessels are distended.
4. Fluids leak out.
5. Inflammation of tissues.
6. Throbbing pain.

Sometimes constriction of the blood vessels for a long time also results in a headache. The mechanism of development of migraine is as shown in Figure 1.

There are several factors that trigger a migraine attack (Box 1). The mechanism of action of common trigger factors are discussed below.

• *Food.* Fasting and missing or delaying a meal can result in a migraine in susceptible people. Foods such as chocolate, cheese, citrus fruits and dairy products can also trigger a migraine. Food can

## Box 1.  Common Migraine Triggers

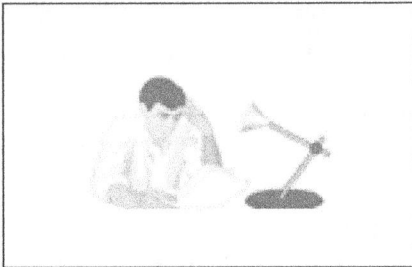

- Fatigue, overwork, travel
- Relaxation after stress
- Bright lights, discos
- Lack of or excess of sleep
- Sensitivity to some foods
- Alcohol, red-wine, icecream
- Menstruation
- Sudden strenuous

cause migraine by three mechanisms: (a) Decrease in blood glucose levels due to lack of food; (b)*"Tyramine"*, a chemical compound found in proteins directly stimulates some cells in the brain. This stimulation constricts the blood vessels of the brain; and (c) Some foods cause allergic reactions. This allergic reaction results in migraine.

Foods rich in tyramine are cheese, beer, red wine, chocolate, beef, liver, canned meats, soy sauce, eggs, broad beans, spinach, oranges, figs, prunes, plums, bananas and tomatoes. Common food allergies in migraine are milk, cheese, tea, coffee, orange juice, tomatoes and potatoes. Some people complain of migraine after eating Chinese food. This is because Chinese food contains a compound called monosodium gluconate. This compound constricts blood vessels of the brain.

Excess of coffee can lead to the headache. On the other hand, people who drink lot of tea, coffee or cola drinks develop headache on sudden withdrawal of caffeine.

Caffeine constricts the blood vessels. Many office going people drink large quantities of tea or coffee at work. During weekends tea and coffee intake may come down. Reduced intake of caffeine causes distension of the blood vessels and therefore headache. This withdrawal headache is usually relieved by drinking tea or coffee.

• *Stress.* Stress is one of the most common causes of migraine. Just like caffeine, stress can cause migraine as soon as it decreases. For example, after working under stress throughout the week if you sleep long hours during weekend, the blood vessels of the brain are distended. Migraine could also be triggered by either excess or lack of sleep, excitement, or physical stress due to jogging or sexual activity. Regular exercise helps control migraine but occasional exercise can lead to a migraine attack.

• *Traveling.* Traveling by any vehicle can lead to migraine mainly due to (a) stress and fatigue; (b) motion sickness; and (c) bright lights at night from vehicles coming from the opposite side.

• *Hormonal changes.* Decreased "*oestrogen*" level in women just before menstruation can trigger a migraine. Women who take contraceptive pills with oestrogen are likely to have very severe migraine.

• **Environmental causes**. Heat, cold, light, noise, or a humid and cloudy weather cause migraine in susceptible people.

• **Anaemia**. It not only results in more severe migraines but also increases the frequency of migraine episodes.

# What are the symptoms of migraine?

Migraine symptoms depend on its type. There are two types of migraine: (1) common migraine; and (2) classical migraine. *Common migraine* is a throbbing pain usually on one side of the head. Pain during each episode lasts for one to three days. This pain is usually associated with nausea, vomiting and increased sensitivity to light and noise. The pain is severe enough to limit your

## Box 2. Symptoms of an aura in migraine

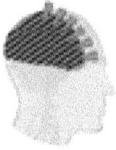

- Focusing problems
- Blind spots in your field of vision
- Coloured lights
- Flashing lines or zigzag
- Hallucinations
- Mood swings
- Speech problems
- Tingling or numbness of hands or face
- Hunger, thirst, food carvings
- Double vision
- Weakness or paralysis on one side of the body

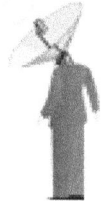

normal activity. The pain in migraine increases by normal physical work. *Classical migraine* is a common migraine plus an "*aura*" before the pain starts. This aura is a warning that a migraine attack is going to start soon. Box 2 lists the common types of aura associated with migraine. A migraine attack has five stages:

• *Prodromal stage.* Nearly fifty percent people who suffer from migraine complain of disturbances in their normal behaviour before an attack. Common disturbances are (i) changes in the mood;

(ii) increased sensitivity to light, noise, smell and touch; (iii) food cravings; and (iv) speech or memory problems. Recognizing prodromal stage is important because medicines taken at this stage can avoid the migraine attack.

• *Aura.* Some people experience an aura about one hour before the headache starts.

• *Headache.* The headache of a migraine is very severe and may last up to seventy-two hours. The muscles in the neck and scalp are painful upon touch. Some people feel better after sleeping for a while in a dark room.

• *Resolution.* In this stage the pain subsides and the body functions return to normal. Resolution can be either a gradual process, as during sleep, or sudden, as after vomiting.

• *Recovery.* Many people feel very tired and drowsy after an attack of migraine. They may also experience mood alterations.

# What is the treatment of migraine?

Four groups of medicines are used to treat migraine. These include:

- analgesics;

- anti-vomiting medicines;

- ergotamine; and

- serotonin stimulants.

- *Analgesics.* Simple analgesics such as paracetamol, aspirin and non-steroidal anti-inflammatory medicines often reduce pain during a migraine attack.

Paracetamol relieves pain. Aspirin and non-steroidal medicines reduce both pain and inflammation.

Common side-effect of aspirin and non-steroidal medicines is irritation of the stomach. This adverse effect is more severe in people with ulcers in the stomach. You should not take these medicines on empty stomach. Stop taking these medicines and consult your doctor immediately if you pass blood in the stool or if the colour of the stool is black. *Aspirin should be avoided in children up to fifteen years and pregnant women*. Non-steroidal anti-inflammatory medicines taken in very large doses for a long time are toxic to liver and kidneys.

• *Anti-vomiting medicines*. Food from the alimentary canal is not absorbed properly during a migraine attack. Anti-vomiting medicines are therefore recommended to: (a) reduce nausea and vomiting; and (b) increase absorption of other medicines. Common types of anti-vomiting medicines used in migraine are metoclopramide and domperidone. These two medicines are often used in combination with other medicines.

• *Ergotamine.* Ergotamine tartarate constricts dilated vessels and dilates constricted vessels. It is most effective if taken early during an attack. Common side effects are nausea, vomiting, and muscle cramps. *Ergotamine should not be taken by pregnant women and patients with heart diseases or diseases of the blood vessels of the hands and legs.*

• *Serotonin stimulants*. These medicines stimulate the serotonin receptors in the brain. Serotonin stimulants reduce inflammation around the blood vessels and constrict the distended blood vessels of the brain. *Sumatriptan*, a serotonin stimulant is the latest medicine used for treatment of migraine attacks. It is used both as an injection and as a tablet. The effect of injection is observed after about half an hour and tablets after about three hours.

Common side effects of sumatriptan are temporary numbness and tingling in the head and neck area; and heaviness and tightness in the chest. These side effects are observed more frequently with injection. *Sumatriptan is not recommended for people suspected of having some heart diseases or uncontrolled high blood pressure. It is also not prescribed for people who are on treatment with ergotamine.* Sumatriptan is the safest medicine currently available for treatment of migraine.

# How can migraine be prevented?

You can prevent frequent episodes of migraine by first identifying the trigger factors and then avoiding them. Trigger factors that you can easily avoid are food, bright lights and irregular strenuous exercise. Some trigger factors, however, are difficult to avoid. These include travel, stress and fatigue. You can prevent frequent attacks of migraine by effectively managing these triggers. For example, regular exercises such as walking and jogging and relaxation techniques such as yoga and meditation are very effective for stress management.

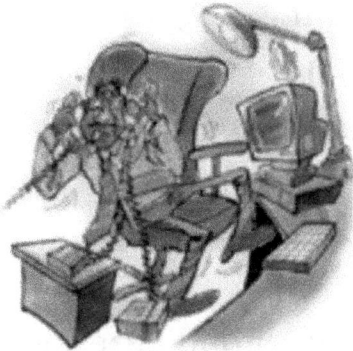

**Why do medicines not cure my headache?**

**Medicines** to prevent migraine attacks are recommended in case you have more than two episodes every month. It may be necessary to take medicines for up to six to eight months. Medicines normally prescribed for prevention of migraine are:

• *Beta-blockers* such as propranolol. Beta-blockers prevent migraine by regulating serotonin levels in the brain. Common side effects are lethargy, lack of motivation, depression, lower levels of blood pressure and slowing of the heart rate.

• *Calcium channel blockers* such as flunarizine and nimodipine. This group of medicines also regulates serotonin levels in the brain. Common side effects are constipation, nausea, weight gain and fatigue. Calcium channel blockers can sometimes cause involuntary muscle movements.

• *Serotonin uptake inhibitors* such as pizotefen and cyprohepatidine. This group of medicines block the receptors for serotonin in the brain. This block prevents distension of blood vessels. Common side effects are drowsiness and increased appetite.

• *Anti-depressants* such as amytryptyline. This group of

medicines prevents migraine by promoting more natural sleep patterns. The dose required to prevent migraines is usually less than that required to control depression. Common side effects are drowsiness, constipation, dry mouth and weight gain.

# Tension Headache

## What is tension headache?

Headache due to contraction of muscles of the neck and head is called tension headache. You can identify painful areas on the muscles on the back of the neck during a tension headache. This is done by running your fingers on any side of the back of the neck, especially from the point where the neck joins the shoulders to the base of your head. More than seventy percent of all headaches are tension headache. This headache is short-lived. In fact many people refer to tension headache as their "normal headache".

# What are the causes of tension headache?

Common causes of the tension headache are emotional stress, overwork, lack of sleep, poor posture, eye strain, and using the neck in an awkward posture. Most people hunch their shoulders and hold them very tightly during stress. You can test this yourself when you are under stress. Observe the position of your shoulders in relation to the neck, shrug your shoulders, hold them for a moment and let them relax consciously. You will notice that your shoulders drop, thus indicating that they were tense before. The neck and shoulder muscles also become tense due to any activity or exercise which requires you to hold your neck bent backwards.

You are likely to tightly screw up your eyes whenever you look at bright lights. This results in contraction of the face muscles and therefore headache. This can also happen if you have poor eyesight and you do not wear corrective glasses regularly.

Bad posture also results in tension headache. Incorrect level or distance of a typewriter or computer is a common cause for this headache. Holding your neck in a wrong position while working on your desk results in contraction of the neck muscles. Contraction of the neck and face muscles and pain often form a vicious cycle. Whenever you have pain due to contraction of these muscles, you are more likely to hold your head very stiff. This results in more prolonged muscle contraction and therefore more pain.

# What are the symptoms of tension headache?.

People with tension headache complain of any one of the following symptoms:

- a feeling of tightness;

- a feeling of heavy weight pressing on the top of the head; or

- a feeling of a tight band around the head and neck. The pain is usually felt all over the head. In some cases it may be located on top of the head. The tension headache is usually present on both sides of the head. These headaches can occur everyday and are normally more severe in the evenings.

• **Vascular headaches**. These headaches spread throughout the head and are throbbing in nature. Causes of vascular headaches are:

• infections;

• reduced oxygen supply to the brain;

• reduced levels of the glucose in the blood;

• alcohol;

• nitrates, which are prescribed for some heart diseases; and

• medicines, such as Histamine antagonists (e.g. Ranitidine) used for gastric ulcer. Fever and sinusitis are common infections associated with the headache.

**Effort induced headaches**. There are three common types of effort that can result in a headache. These are:

• *Benign exertional headache*. This type of headache is mainly observed in men. The pain starts at the end of sudden vigorous exercise such as running. It may resemble migraine. In susceptible people, it can also lead to a migraine.

- *Cough headache.* Coughing, straining or lifting weight often result in the headache.

- *Coital headache.* Some people may have headache after sexual intercourse. Cough and coital headache need to be distinguished from more serious cause of headache.

# Management of an episode of tension headache

The following are simple but effective way to manage a tension headache.

• Apply wet heat to head and neck (such as hot showers) two to three times a day.

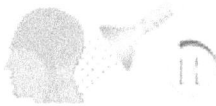

• Massage the back of the neck and shoulders. Most commercial massage cream relax muscles.

They contain menthol or peppermint oil

• Take a mild analgesic such as paracetamol or aspirin. Remember not to make it a habit of taking them

• Do some simple exercise such as walking or jogging. Yoga, meditation and relaxation methods are effective

# What are the serious causes of headache?

Sub-arachnoid haemorrhage (bleeding in the space around the brain); meningitis (brain fever); increased pressure on the brain; severe hypertension; and temporal arteritis are some of the serious causes of headache. You should consult with a doctor in a major hospital immediately for these causes.

# Indications for specialist consultation and investigations in headache

One should consult a specialist and go for indepth investigations of the following symptoms are noticed.

• A first attack of severe headache — 'worst ever headache' in one's life.

• Recent onset or long lasting and progressively increasing headaches. More so when accompanied with blurring of vision, deteriorating memory, social-withdrawal of a part of body, epileptic attacks.

• Headache accompanied with

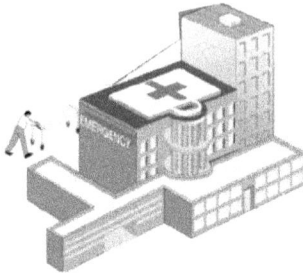

fever and neck pain with stiff neck.

• Headache in a drowsy or confused person, with abnormal physical signs. Headache heralded by physical exertion.

# What is sub-arachnoid haemorrhage?

The brain is covered by three thin layers of tissue. "*Arachnoid*" is the middle layer of the tissue. Main blood vessels supplying blood to the brain run between the arachnoid and the third layer of the brain. If one of these blood vessels bursts, blood is released into the gap between the arachnoid and the brain. Since the brain is located inside a bony cage, the blood cannot expand outside.

Thus, the haemorrhage pushes the soft tissue of the brain inside and raises the pressure inside the head.

Spontaneous sub-arachnoid haemorrhage occurs in patients with weakness in the walls of the blood vessels of the brain and some heart diseases. The blood vessels of the brain often burst during straining, sexual activity, forced evacuation of stools and after head injury. The impact of sub-arachnoid haemorrhage is dramatic. Within seconds the affected person gets very severe headache and becomes unconscious. The symptoms depend upon the site of haemorrhage and the amount of bleeding. If the bleeding is not very severe, the person will complain of very severe headache, will be either drowsy or irritable, and will have altered consciousness. People with mild bleeding often say that they had a feeling of being hit on the back of the head followed by severe headache.

Sub-arachnoid haemorrhage is a medical emergency. *Immediate* admission to a major hospital is necessary. Recovery depends upon: (a) the amount of bleeding; and (b) the time lag between bleeding and starting the treatment. It may take a long time and may not be complete. It is important to know that this type of haemorrhage is very rare. It occurs more often among people with high blood pressure. Maintaining normal blood pressure greatly reduces the risk of haemorrhage.

# What is meningitis?

Meningitis is the infection of the loose coverings of the brain called the *"meninges"*. The brain floats in a fluid called the *"cerebro-spinal fluid"*. This fluid supports the brain and protects it from shocks. Sometimes the meninges get infected and start producing pus. This pus is full of bacteria. It directly enters the cerebro-spinal fluid in which the brain floats. The bacteria and viruses come in direct contact with the brain and infect it very quickly.

The common symptoms of meningitis are fever, headache, stiffness of the neck and vomiting. The patient cannot tolerate light and soon becomes drowsy or unconsciousness. Anyone who has fever and stiff neck should be rushed to a major hospital immediately. The faster the treatment starts, greater are the chances of recovery. Delayed treatment often results in death.

# How does tension headache differ from migraine?

The tension headache differs from migraine in four ways. In tension headache

- you can continue doing your work during headache;

- there is no increase in severity of pain due to normal work and physical activity;

- there are no associated symptoms such as nausea,

vomiting, intolerance to light and sound; and

- there is no disturbance in the sleep.

# What is the treatment of tension headache?

Tension headache can be cured by medicines and non-medicine measures. *Medicines* are of limited use in this type of headache. Many people take simple pain killers. Pain killers reduce just the pain and therefore give relief for some time. When the effect of the medicine wears off, the headache returns. This is because muscle contraction is still there. As the severity of the pain increases, the medicines which do not relax the muscles become less effective. In fact many people with regular tension headaches get very worried because the pain does not go away with simple pain killers. They begin to believe that their headache could be because of some serious problems.

People who take regular habit-forming medicines are likely to suffer from headaches when they stop taking these medicines. Medicines that result in this type of rebound headache are analgesics, tranquilizers and sedatives.

Aspirin or paracetamol and amytryptyline are commonly used for tension headache.

**Non-medicinal measures** are very effective for control of tension headache. Management of an episode of tension headache is described in an earlier chapter. However, long-term benefit is possible if you identify events that bring a headache and manage them effectively. Very often, you may either not remember these events, or not even be aware of them. Therefore, every time you get a headache, try to identify the cause and write it in a diary. Review of these causes of headache over a period of time will help you to understand the type of emotional, psychological and physical stress that results in a headache. You should also try to correct other causes of tension headache, if any. These include wearing correct glasses if you have poor vision, treatment from a dentist to improve the way you bite food; and regular exercises for cervical spondylosis.

*Regular exercise and relaxation techniques* such as yoga and meditation are useful for managing stress. Effective stress management reduces the frequency of tension headaches. If you are not able to deal with stress through regular exercise and relaxation techniques, you may need to consult a mental health specialist who will help you manage the stress. Some people with latent depression complain of tension headache. They also have disturbed sleep early in the morning, mood swings and negative attitude towards life. Their headache is more severe in the morning. Treatment by mental health specialist is necessary for managing headache of people with latent depression. Majority of these people respond very well to short-term treatment.

# Cluster Headache

## What is cluster headache?

Cluster headache is a group of symptoms. It affects men about six times more frequently than women. The episodes usually start after twenty years of age. They are observed more frequently among those who smoke and consume alcohol. Each headache episode may last from fifteen minutes to three hours. Many such episodes may occur during a day and last for several weeks. The pain starts behind or around one eye. There is no associated aura. Many people get up from their sleep due to severe pain.

## How can you diagnose a cluster headache?

A person with cluster headache will have at least five attacks fulfilling the following criteria:

• Very severe pain around or above any one eye. May have pain above the ears also. Each episode lasts for 15-180 minutes without treatment.

• Headache is associated with at least one of these: Conjunctivitis, increased water secretion from the eyes, congestion of the nose,

running nose, swelling of forehead

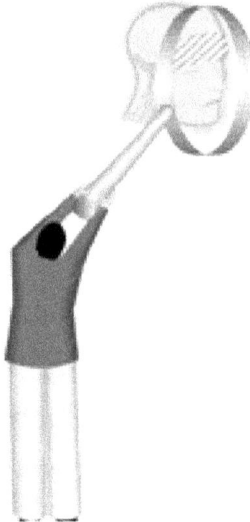

and face, very small pupils, drooping of one or both eyelids, swelling of the eyelids.

- Frequency of attacks: once in two days to eight times a day.

History and physical examination of not suggest any brain disorders with head injury.

**Treatment** of cluster headache aims at prevention of the attacks. Since the headache comes for several days around the same time of the day, it is possible to prevent these headaches by taking timely medicine. *Ergotamine* is usually given one hour before the expected attack. Other medicines recommended are sumatriptan, calcium channel blockers such as verapamil, and methysergide. Indomethacin is recommended if the episodes are very frequent. Occasionally your doctor may recommend "*steroids*" to control recurrent attacks of cluster headache. Steroids should be taken only under direct supervision of the doctor.

# What are other common causes of headache?

**Cervicogenic headache**. This type of headache is due to cervical spondylosis. Cervical spondylosis is a degenerative condition of the neck. People who suffer from cervical spondylosis often have pain on one or both sides of the neck due to muscle contraction. The pain spreads to the base of the head, just above the ears and also the forehead. The pain lasts throughout the day. It increases with neck movements. Proper exercises that relax the muscles of the back of the neck and head prevent this type of headache. Applying heat to the back of the neck also relaxes the muscles.

**Headache after injury**. Even a minor injury to the head causes severe headache. This is mainly due:

• to local bruise of the skin and muscles of the scalp; and

• stretching of the nerves in the scalp. Minor injuries also result in contraction of the muscles of the head and neck.

**Vascular headaches**. These headaches spread throughout the head and are throbbing in nature. Causes of vascular headaches are:

- infections;

- reduced oxygen supply to the brain;

- reduced levels of the glucose in the blood;

- alcohol;

- nitrates, which are prescribed for some heart diseases; and

- medicines, such as Histamine antagonists (e.g. Ranitidine) used for gastric ulcer. Fever and sinusitis are common infections associated with the headache.

**Effort induced headaches**. There are three common types of effort that can result in a headache. They are:

• *Benign exertional headache*. This type of headache is mainly observed in men. The pain starts at the end of sudden vigorous exercise such as running. It may resemble migraine. In susceptible people, it can also lead to a migraine.

• *Cough headache*. Coughing, straining or lifting weights often result in the headache.

• *Coital headache*. Some people may have headache after sexual intercourse. Cough and coital headaches need to be distinguished from more serious causes of headache.

# What are the causes of increased pressure on the brain?

A tumor, abscess, or chronic inflammatory mass such as the *"Tuberculoma"* are the common causes of increased pressure of the brain. They may not cause headaches in the early stages. Very often the headache is observed only after more serious complications such as paralysis. Any tumor that grows inside the skull puts pressure on the brain at the site of its growth. It also stops the outflow of the cerebro-spinal fluid and therefore raises pressure within the skull. A rise in the pressure causes dull persistent headaches.

# What is temporal arteritis?

The *temple* is the region between and just above your eyes and ears. The artery which runs across the temple on both sides is called temporal artery. Rarely, there is inflammation of the tissues inside this artery. This condition is called temporal arteritis. It is not a common disease but if not treated, can cause blindness almost overnight. It can also reduce blood supply to part of the brain and result in a "*stroke*".

Temporal arteritis is mainly observed in people above fifty years. Any new headache in the temple in elderly people should be investigated for temporal arteritis. The artery is sometimes prominent and painful to touch. If the doctor suspects temporal arteritis, he will ask you to undertake a blood test called the *"Erythrocyte Sedimentation Rate"* (ESR). An ESR reading more than fifty millimeters in the first one hour indicates temporal arteritis. The doctor may also remove a small piece of the artery and examine it under the microscope. This test is called a *"biopsy"*. This is the confirmative test for temporal arteritis.

Steroids are the only medicines recommended for treatment of temporal arteritis. They reduce headaches rapidly and there is no further risk of loosing eyesight. You may have to take steroids for a very long time - sometimes even throughout life. Your doctor will initially recommend very high doses of steroids. He will also regularly monitor you ESR readings. As the ESR readings come down, he will gradually reduce the steroid dose. *It is important to remember that you should never stop steroids suddenly. You should reduce the dose very slowly and only under the direct supervision of your doctor.*

# AYURVEDA

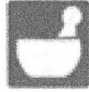

The Ayurveda system of medicine describes three broad categories of the diseases of the brain. These include: *shirashula, shirobhitapa and shirovedana.* The type of headache in these diseases is piercing, burning and dull headache respectively.

# What are the causes of headache?

Causes of the diseases of the brain are broadly divided into six groups. These include:

• *Diet (Aharajanya)*. Excessive intake of heavy and sour articles and greens, and drinking very cold water are common causes of headache. Poor digestion of food results in semi-fluid mass of partly digested food expelled into the food pipe above also results in headache.

• *Life-style    (Viharajanya).* Suppression of natural desires, sleeping during the day time, inadequate sleep at night, alcohol intake, talking very loudly, exposure to cold weather

• especially at night and excess of sexual act are common causes of headache.

• *Environment (Asatmyajanya).* Unpleasant smell, facing head-winds, and exposure to dust, smoke, cold and heat can also cause headache.

• *Psychological (Manojanya).* Psychological stress, excessive crying or suppression of tears can lead to headache.

• *Season (Ritujanya).* Some people have headache when there is abnormality in notmal climate or season, or just before the onset of rains.

• *Injury (Abhighatajanya).* Any injury to the head, irrespective of its severity, can cause headache.

# What is the *Tridosha* theory for headache?

According to the basic principles of Ayurveda there are three *doshas* in the body. They are *Vata, pitta and kapha*. Doshas do not have an English equivalent. Together these three doshas are known as *tridoshas*.

Vata is responsible for movement and sensation within the cell and the whole body. It is formed with two elements of the universe — ether and air. Pitta is

## Fig 2. Ayurvedic philosophy of mechanism of development of ache

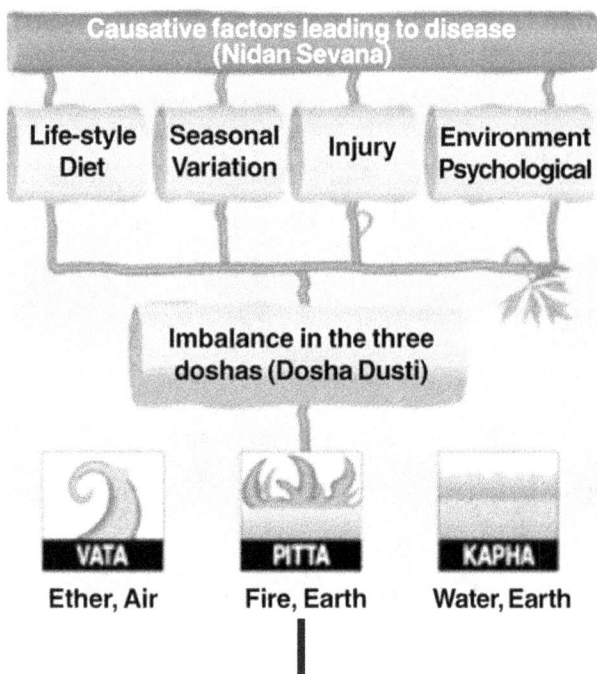

Causative factors leading to disease (Nidan Sevana)

| Life-style Diet | Seasonal Variation | Injury | Environment Psychological |

Imbalance in the three doshas (Dosha Dusti)

| VATA | PITTA | KAPHA |
| Ether, Air | Fire, Earth | Water, Earth |

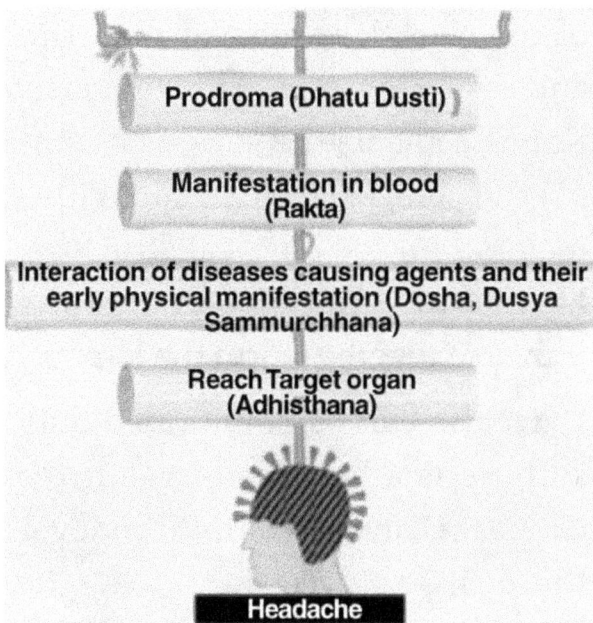

Prodroma (Dhatu Dusti)

Manifestation in blood (Rakta)

Interaction of diseases causing agents and their early physical manifestation (Dosha, Dusya Sammurchhana)

Reach Target organ (Adhisthana)

Headache

the heat and energy in the body. It is responsible for digestion, absorption, assimilation, nutrition, metabolism, skin colour and lustre of the eyes. It is formed with fire and earth elements of the universe. Kapha cements the various organs of the body. It also provides material for the physical structure. Earth and water elements of the universe together form the kapha.

Health can be maintained only if there is a balance of the three doshas. Disease results whenever there is an imbalance in the proportion of these doshas. This imbalance can also result in headache. Figure 2 describes the mechanism of developing headache.

*Charaka,* the famous physician who lived sometime between the second century BC and the second century AD, has mentioned several diseases under the category of diseases of the head. These include:

- pain in one side of the head;

- diffused pain of the entire head;

- upper respiratory tract infection;

- diseases of the nose, eyes, and ears;

- giddiness;

- loss of sensation and motility (paralysis) of the face;

- tremors of the head;

- contraction of the throat, neck and jaws;

- other diseases resulting from imbalances in the *doshas;* and

- parasitic infections.

# What is the treatment of headache?

The treatment of headache depends upon the cause of headache. Various types of remedies recommended in Ayurveda include

- single drug therapy;
- nasal instillation;
- local applications;
- decoctions; and
- herbo-mineral combinations
- animal fat based preparations; and

- medicated oils.

  **Single drug therapy** includes:

- *Local application of Muchukunda flowers.* A paste prepared from these flowers should be applied to the head for relief of headache. These flowers are useful both in one-sided pain and diffused pain throughout the head. It reduces vata in the body and thus restores the balance of tridoshas.

- *Powdered preparation from Rauvolfia serpentina.* This medicinal plant has been used extensively for treatment of high blood pressure. In addition, the powdered preparation of this plant relieves the piercing type of headache if taken with honey three times a day.

• *Godhanti bhasma* or hydrated calcium sulfate. Taking it with honey three times a day in a dose recommended by your doctor relieves the dull type of headache.

• *Local application of costus or kuth.* A paste is prepared from the root of the plant with castor oil. It reduces *vata* and reduces piercing type of headache.

Ayurveda also recommends wearing a cap filled with medicinal preparations for relief from headache.

**Nasal instillation** commonly used for treatment of headache clear passages in and around the nose and increase circulation of the blood in the head. Cleared passages and increased blood circulation relieves headache by removing toxic matter. Powdered bark of bay berry and *ghee* instillation are recommended for relief of migraine. *Shad bindu tail* and *Anu tail* give relief from headache due to sinusitis. Instillation of milk and extract of the sacred *kusagrass* have been observed to abort an attack of migraine if taken in the prodromal stage. They also give relief in dull headaches.

**Local applications** of a combination of medicinal herbs reduces *vata* which is the root cause of pain. There are more than a dozen preparations recommended in Ayurveda for various causes of the headache. Some of the commonly used prescriptions are:

• a paste of the bark of conifers or pine, East Indian rosebay, musk root, and dried ginger prepared in a fermented substance called *Kanji;*

• a paste of long-pepper, liquorice, *nagar motha*, aniseed, Indian water lily, and costus root prepared in water;

• a paste of black gingelly, and nardus root prepared in a rock salt and honey; and

• a paste of wild asparagus, gingelly, liquorice, and Indian water lily.

**Decoction** of fruits of chebulic myrobalan and nine other herbs is very useful for piercing type of headache. Similarly, decoction prepared mainly from long and round pepper is also recommended for piercing type of the headaches. These decoctions should be taken for three to

four days.

**Herbo-mineral** preparations recommended in Ayurveda relax constricted blood vessels of the brain. Most of these preparations need to be taken twice a day for five to seven days. Herbo-mineral preparations are not recommended for people with diseases of the kidneys. Commonly used preparations are:

- *Sirah suladri vajra rasa.* This is a preparation of four minerals and twenty herbs. It is one of the most commonly used preparations for control of all headaches.

- *Mahalakshmi vilas rasa.* This is a preparation of two minerals and fifteen herbs. It is particularly recommended for headaches due to common cold or dull type of headache.

• *Tribhuvana kirti rasa.* This preparation is very effective for control of migraine.

• *Chandramrita rasa.* This preparation of seven minerals and thirteen herbs relieves pain of all types of headache.

In addition to the above therapies, some medicated oils are also recommended for local application and massage. Massage with these oils relaxes muscles of the head and neck.

# What is the recommended diet during headache?

Consumption of red variety of rice, vegetable soup, milk, *patola* (a vegetable), drumstick, grapes, pomegranate, curd or yogurt prepared from skim milk and tender coconut water are recommended during an attack of headache.

# What are the aggravating factors?

Consumption of contaminated water, food you are allergic to and cold drinks can aggravate the headache. Similarly over-eating can also increase the intensity of the pain. Other factors that can aggravate the headache are:

- suppression of natural urges;
- sleeping during the day;
- consumption of alcohol;
- lack of sleep at night; and
- excessive sex.

# HOMOEOPATHY

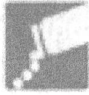

The Homoeopathic system of medicine also recognizes headache as a universal experience. It can either be simple pain or heaviness in the head, and it can be a very severe or persistent pain. The causes and types of headache described in this system of medicine are the same as discussed in the section on Allopathy. The causes can be summarized into two broad categories:

## Box 3. Site of pain for various causes of headache

### Front of the head

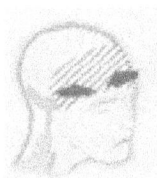

Tension headache

Toothache

Sinusitus

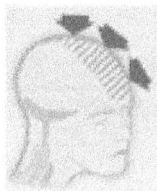

**Sides of the head**

Tension headache

Migraine

Temporal arteritis

**Middle or all over**

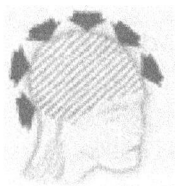

Tension headache

Tumor

## Back of the head and/or neck

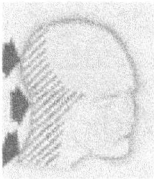

Tension headache

Meningitis •

Subarachnoid
haemorrhage •

Cervical spondylosis

**Around/above the eyes**

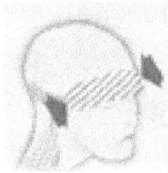

Tension headache

Migraine

Cluster headache

- Requires immediate medical help

- headache due to causes outside the brain. These include sinusitis, diseases of the eyes, toothache, cervical spondylosis, temporal arteritis and stretching and contraction of the muscles and blood vessels in the neck and scalp;

- headache due to causes inside the brain. These include brain tumors, bleeding in the space around the brain and high blood pressure.

*Homoeopathy medicines are very effective for treatment of migraine (although it takes some time for complete cure); and headache as a result of emotional stress, grief, fear, remorse, and injury to the head. They are also very effective in headaches due to sinusitis.*

# What is the treatment of headache?

There are no conventional pain-killers in Homoeopathy. However, there are more than three hundred Homoeopathic medicines for treatment of headache. Selection of medicines will depend on the condition of your headache and the combination of symptoms you may have. If you do not describe all the symptoms to the doctor, he/she may not be able to prescribe the correct medicines. Your detailed history will also determine the course of your headaches and other additional therapy the doctor may need to prescribe. *It is therefore important that you* explain at least the following four conditions to the doctor:

- cause of your headache

- other associated symptoms, **even if you think they are not important or not related to the headache**;

- *factors that increase or decrease the pain; and*

- *other symptoms after the headache starts.*

Homoeopathic medicines are different for various causes of headache. For example, different medicines are prescribed for the headaches due to shock, mental exhaustion, depression, anger, crying, migraines, injury and left- or right-sided headaches. Medicines control the basic cause of the headache and therefore relieve you of the pain.

Your doctor may recommend that you keep some medicines at home for use during times when it is not possible to go to the doctor immediately. These medicines will help till you are able to consult with your doctor. Medicines that you can keep at home include:

• *Ignatia and Natrum Mur*. These are very effective in controlling headache due to emotional causes such as grief. They should be taken three to four times a day till the symptoms subside.

• *Aconite* is an effective medicine if you have headache due to fear.

• *Arnica.* This is an extremely effective medicine for controlling headache due to injury. Take this medicine as soon as you have either minor or severe injury to the head. You can repeat the medicine every three hours until you are able to consult with a doctor. Other medicines that may be recommended by your doctor are Natrum Mur., Natrum Sulph and Cicuta.

# What is the mechanism of action of Homoeopathic medicines?

All Homoeopathic medicines are absorbed from the mucous membrane of the tongue. They send messages to the brain through the nerve endings in the tongue. These medicines enhance your body's natural healing mechanisms. Most medicines used for treatment of headache increase secretion of *endorphins*. Endorphins are chemical substances secreted by the brain. They are natural pain killers.

# How long should the medicines be taken?

Initially, the medicines reduce acute pain within ten to fifteen minutes. These medicines are repeated every two to three hours till the acute pain subsides. Subsequently, the Homoeopathic medicines cure, or at least control the cause(s) of the headache. It may be necessary to take these medicines for several days, weeks or months. Duration of treatment is reduced by regular intake of medicines and changes in the life-style as recommended by your doctor. Most Homoeopathic medicines for treatment of the headaches do not have any side effects or aggravation of symptoms. However, some people may have drowsiness, diarrhoea and vomiting for a few hours.

## How are frequent episodes of the headache prevented?

Regular exercise, yoga, meditation and other similar relaxation techniques help control frequent attacks of the headaches. These measures reduce stress and relax the muscles of the head and neck, thus preventing headaches. They also increase your threshold of tolerance to the physical and emotional stress. You should also eat plenty of fresh fruits and raw vegetables. These foods regulate your bowel movements and therefore help control the headaches.

# What are the limitations of Homoeopathic medicines for controlling headaches?

• Homoeopathic medicines cannot cure the headaches for those who are not willing to change their life-style such as high intake of alcohol, irregular sleep and dietary habits.

• Homoeopathic medicines are not effective for serious causes of headache such as brain tumor.

• Some people on regular Allopathic treatment for diseases

such as hypertension, diabetes, etc. complain of frequent headaches. Homoeopathic medicines may not be able to completely cure their headaches.

# NATURE CURE

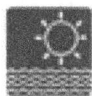

Causes and types of the headache described in Nature Cure are the same as those described in the section on Allopathy. This system also emphasizes the importance of suitable life-styles for prevention and control of the headaches. It believes that faulty attitude towards nature and its principle disturbs the digestive system. This disturbance results in formation of gases and acids. These gases enter the blood and irritate various cells including the nerve cells. Irritation of nerve cells causes headaches.

# What is the treatment for headache?

Nature Cure treatment for the headaches depends upon its cause. Detailed below are the management options for common causes of headache.

**Headache due to indigestion.** Disturbances of the digestive system results in many diseases. Headache is one of them. Thus, a healthy digestive system will have other benefits also. The following measures help to maintain a healthy digestive system by preventing gas formation:

• *Drinking at least eight to ten glasses of water* every day. You should drink one glass of water every two hours. You should also drink three to four glasses of water on empty stomach as soon as you get up. This helps to activate your bowel movements.

• *Passing stools every morning* **and** *evening*. You should train your body to evacuate twice a day. This will prevent formation of gases from undigested food.

• *Abdominal pack.* Three hours after every dinner, keep a cloth dipped in cold water on the abdomen for twenty minutes. This abdominal pack will increase blood circulation of various organs in your abdomen. Increased circulation improves digestion.

• *Enema.* A warm water enema is recommended if you suffer from constipation. You should evacuate after five to ten minutes of taking the enema.

**Headache due to nervous tension**. Physical and mental stress results in tightening of muscles of the head and neck. This tightening results in the headache. The following measures help relax your head and neck muscles:

• Stretching of the neck and shoulders relieves pain.

• Massaging the head, neck and shoulders.

• Keeping a hot water bag or heating pad on the neck. Heat increases the blood circulation and therefore relaxes the muscles.

• Pouring hot and cold water on the neck alternately also results in increased blood circulation. This results in relaxation of muscles.

• Keeping your backbone in contact with cold water in a special spinal bath tub for thirty minutes relaxes the mind. A relaxed mind helps control the headaches.

**Headache caused due to cold and other respiratory complaints.** Colds and other respiratory infections result in congestion of the nose and respiratory tract. This congestion can cause headache. The following measures are recommended for reducing the congestion of the respiratory tract:

• *Hot foot bath*. In this bath, you should keep your legs up to knees in a bucket of hot water. Your body should be covered with a blanket to prevent loss of body heat. The head should be covered with a cold cloth. A hot foot bath for five to twenty minutes helps control the headaches in three ways: (a) it increases bowel movements; (b) relieves congestion due to cold; and (c) constricts dilated blood vessels of the brain. It is important to remember that you should drink at least one glass of water before taking this bath.

• *Steam inhalation*. Inhaling steam increases blood circulation

## Box 4. You and your headache

- Do not brood over simple headache which often are due to tension migraine or referred from near by structures like air filled sinuses around the nose and eyes or tooth and gums.

- Serious headache are only 1% of all headaches; do not worry about you developing serious diseases such as brain tumour.

- Do not self medicate.

- Your doctor is the best person to decide what type of headache you are suffering from.

144

of the head and the respiratory organs. It also opens up the nasal passages. Increased blood circulation and open nasal passages reduce the congestion.

• *Steam bath.* In this bath, the Nature Cure doctor will ask you to sit in a special cabinet for ten to twenty minutes. This will result in a lot of sweating. Increased sweating removes waste matter in your body. You should have a cold water bath immediately after the steam bath. Alternative steam and cold bath increases blood circulation. You should drink one or two glasses of cold water before taking the steam bath and cover your head with a cold towel.

*Pregnant women, and those with heart diseases or high blood pressure should not take this bath. It is important to remember that if you feel tired or uncomfortable during the bath, you should come out of the steam cabinet immediately and drink cold water.*

**Headache caused due to food.** Some people develop headache after eating foods like ice-cream, tomatoes, cheese, Chinese foods, etc. You should learn to identify foods that result in the headaches and avoid them. If your headache is because you have stopped drinking tea or coffee or smoking, keep a cold compress on the head and sleep for a while in a dark room. Cold compress will constrict distended blood vessels of the brain. Sleeping in a dark room will help you relax.

**Migraine**. The following measures should be taken as soon as you get migraine. These measures reduce distention of the blood vessels of the brain.

• Vomiting after taking four to five glasses of luke warm water with salt.

• Hot foot bath.

• Enema.

• Drink large quantities of warm water till the headache comes down. You can also take hot honey water or vegetable soups.

• Massage head and muscles of the leg below the knees.

**Diet**. High fibre diet improves bowel movements. It also helps complete evacuation of stools. Thus there will be no acid and gas formation in the digestive system.

148

You should eat regular meals consisting of whole cereals, nuts, fruits, leafy vegetables, legumes and tubers. Avoid milk and milk products as they can trigger migraine headaches. Citrus fruits

**?**

**Do You Know That**

Most structures in the brain are not sensitive to pain. Blood vessels inside and outside the body cage of the head are sensitive to pain. Their distension, distortion and inflammation is felt as pain.

and their juices remove toxins from the body. Removal of toxins often helps control the headaches. However, you should avoid citrous fruits if you have migraine headaches.

Eating soaked prunes early in the morning and after dinner prevents constipation.

A dressing with onion or cabbage applied on the back of the neck, calf muscles and soles of the feet constricts distended blood vessels of the brain during the headaches.

# HEALTH TIP

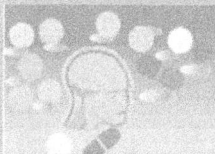

Taking medicine in anticipation of tension headache worsens the problem. It leads to dependence on medicines and more frequent headaches. You are, therefore, advised not to take medicines without your doctor's recommendation.

# Definitions

*Arachnoid* is a thin, delicate membrane that covers the brain and the spinal cord. It lies in between two other coverings of the brain and spinal cord.

*Biopsy* is removal of a small piece of living tissue from any organ or part of the body. This part is examined under a microscope for making diagnosis.

*Cerebro-spinal fluid* is the fluid that flows through and around the brain. It protects the brain from shocks.

*Erythrocyte-sedimentation rate* is the rate at which red blood cells settle out in a tube of blood that is not clotted. It is expressed in millimeters per hour.

*Estrogen* is one of the hormones, a chemical substance, that promotes development of female secondary sex characteristics.

*Hereditary factors* are factors that are transmitted from one generation to the other.

*Meninges* are any one of the three membranes that cover the brain and the spinal cord.

*Receptor* in the context of the headache refers to the nerve ending which responds to various stimuli.

*Serotonin* is a chemical substance found in the brain, intestines and some blood cells. It pays a crucial role in transmission of messages through the nerves.

*Steroids* are a group of chemical substances similar to those secreted by some organs of the body. They are used for treatment of many diseases such as asthma, skin disorders, etc.

*Stroke* is a condition where either there is rupture or obstruction of a blood vessel of the brain. It may lead to sudden paralysis and/or decrease or loss of consciousness.

*Tuberculoma* is a growth on the brain or spinal cord caused by the bacteria that causes tuberculosis.

*Tyramine* is chemical substance found in proteins. It stimulates the adrenal gland to release certain chemical substances which constrict the blood vessels.

# References

## Allopathy

Adams R.D. Principles of Neurology, 1993

Caplan L.R. Consultation in Neurology, 1988

Couch T.R. 'Headache to worry about' in Medical Clinics of North America; 1993 : 77; 141-163

Edmeads J. Postgraduate Medicine, 1989,86;93-110

Neurology : 1993, 43 (supplement 3) : S11-S15

Pearce J.M.S.    N e u r o l o g i c a l
disorders, 1995

Progression clinical Neuroscience -
1991,7:121-135    (published    by
Neurology Society of India

**Ayurveda**

Charaka Samhita

Susruta Samhita

Astanga Hridaya

Chakradutta

Bhaishjya Ratnavali

A   hand   book   of   Domestic
Medicines    and    Common
Ayurvedic Remedies, published
by Central

Council for Research in Ayurveda and Siddha, New Delhi.

Bhava Prakasha

Vangasena

Madhava Nidana

Madhava Chikitsa

**Homoeopathy**

Speight Phyllis, A comparism of the chronic miasms.

Banerjee P.N., Chronic Diseases.

Vithoulkas George Dr., Homoeopathy - Medicine of the New Man.

Boericke William Dr., Homoeopathic Materia Medica.

Kanjilal J.N., Writings on Homoeopathy.

Mazumdar K.P. Dr., Lectures on Homoeopathic Therapeutics.

**Nature Cure**

Vogel A. Swiss, Nature Doctor

Burkitt Denes Dr., Don't forget fibre in your diet.

Murphy Wendy, Dealing with headaches.